I Have Breast Cancer, Now What?

A Cancer Support Tool

Natalie K. Smalley

I have Breast Cancer, Now What?
A Cancer Support Tool

CONTENTS

FOREWORD

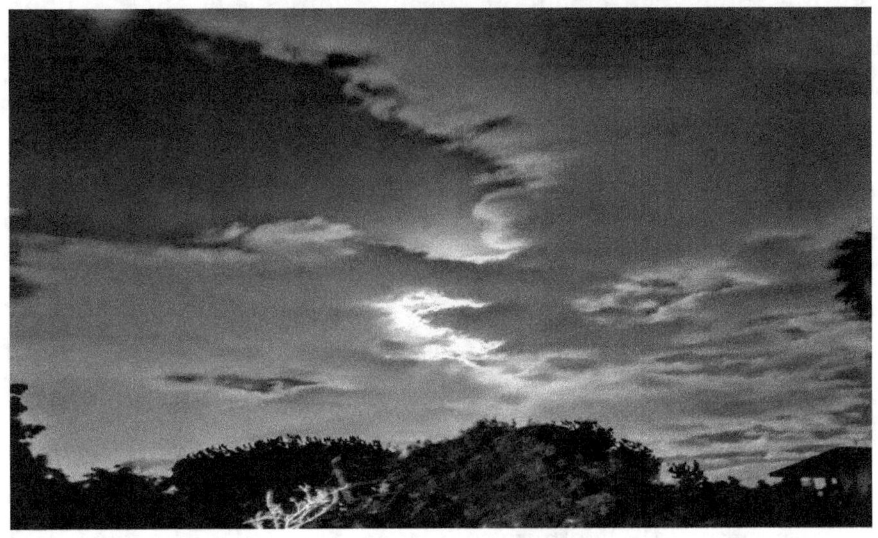

Hello, and thank you for joining me for this book. I am humbled and honored to share with you some of my real-life experiences with breast cancer and the mastectomy process. I am forever grateful to my standout medical team, leaders, facilitators, health coaches, embracers, supporters, and volunteers that have helped me through my journey.

I am a woman of faith! I was raised in a home that trusted in a faithful God and a God that is a place of security and comfort. I was raised to believe that God is good, and I have always upheld that belief system, even when life got rough. I was still a woman of faith when I heard those words that would change my life forever:

"You have breast cancer!"

I never thought I would hear those words. Sure, I knew that people got cancer, but *me*? And yet, as I heard those words, telling me I had breast cancer, I remained firm in my beliefs. I realized that, while God is my source, I needed access to resources as well. I hope this book can be a positive resource for you, your loved ones, or friends during the cancer journey.

For me, I joined a tremendous organization called Cancer Support Community Pasadena, in my home community of Pasadena, California. I was asked to speak on a few occasions and the delightful experience itself, being able to influence other people and show them this journey is not as insurmountable as it may initially seem, has inspired me to write this book about my journey to reach out to others around the world. No person should have to feel like they have to go through battling breast cancer alone. I will provide resources and contact information at the end of this book to support anyone in need. Now, let's get into a bit about my story.

They say that with cancer, there is Life before Cancer, and then there is Life after Cancer. My last moments of Life before Cancer were in the summer of 2013. Nothing could have prepared me for what I was about to face—I never knew that, as my youngest was preparing to enter his sophomore year of high school, that life would never be the same.

I came home one evening from a day full of activity. I settled in for the night, and as my right arm rubbed up against my right breast, I noticed that it hurt. I tried to brush it off, but the next morning, when I woke up, I noticed spots of blood on my nightgown. Concerned, especially considering the pain I felt the night before, I called my doctor's office, and the nurse on the line quickly scheduled an appointment to check everything out. They found I had infection and inflammation of the breast. The first line of attack was simple—clear out the infection with antibiotics and let the inflammation go down. The plan was to clear it out and then make sure there was no more spotting. As my appointment got closer after a few weeks of letting the medication do its work, I was breathing easily—"Yes!" I told myself. I had no other signs of spotting.

That Sunday, the day before my follow up appointment, I woke up to more spotting of blood. And the next day, I got the confirmation. I had early-stage breast cancer—Ductal Carcinoma in Situ, also known as DCIS. I remember locking arms with my husband after the news, telling him that all I wanted to do was to go to church to pray, and then head to Starbucks for my favorite—a Soy Chai Tea Latte, extra hot.

We decided not to share with the family until we knew more. After all, this was new territory! We met with my Oncologist within the week. The only treatment I was offered was a mastectomy! It was devastating! It shook my whole world! Both my husband and I asked, "Can't you prescribe some kind of medicine? This seems so extreme!" We knew nothing about this world and what we were walking into.

It took a few weeks to come to terms with what had to happen. According to my doctors, my left breast was pristine. It was spotless, and though we asked, not necessary to consider removing as well. So, supported by my husband, our Smalley-Bunch of eight children, other family, and friends, I was prepped for the surgery. Further consultation with my Plastic Surgeon confirmed that the process of reconstruction, which I chose, could begin during the mastectomy surgery. This meant the insertion of a breast expander, which ultimately would stretch the skin and prepare my body for silicone implants. Post-surgery and recovery were challenging, but my doctor was encouraging to the end. She asked me to look at my recovery as I would a marathon race as opposed to a sprint.

After months of leave from work, I came back with a new lease on life! I got involved in Toast Masters. I revisited Voice Over classes that opened the door for me at Pacifica's KPFK Radio.org. And I continued to walk in faith and hope to the best of my ability. It wasn't easy by any means, but I did it.

Fast forward to 2016—my left side was due for a mammogram. We had been busy planning our travel with our youngest son to Greenville, IL, for his first year of college. I received a phone call in the midst of preparations that informed me that my mammogram had to be repeated. There was calcification present. It was a common occurrence, and very small, but given my history of past breast cancer, they wanted to ensure that it was nothing dangerous.

We couldn't believe what was happening—the results would be ready while we were in Illinois. We had said our goodbyes to our last college freshman. As we were singing the praises of being empty nesters, driving down a 2-lane highway in the Midwest with beautiful picturesque open-field countryside the call came in. We had to pull over. That pristine and spotless left breast that had been spared was now infected by this dark disease. It was a different cancer this time—I had the option of either a lumpectomy or a mastectomy. I chose the latter.

This meant war!! We felt like this time; we knew what we were dealing with; it wasn't our first rodeo, but I couldn't see myself going through this again. I felt lost! I felt betrayed! Why was this happening again? How could we possibly get through it again?

I felt like I needed more this time. I remembered the Kaiser Hospital Breast Cancer Coordinator telling me about a support group—the Cancer Support Community Pasadena (CSCP). I hadn't checked it out at that point, but when I attended the SoCal Women's Health

Conference and Expo that year, I found myself at a seminar led by Laura Wending, Program Director at the time. She shared her own story and mentioned there were support groups for various cancer situations, classes, and a very specific Lunch Bunch group with others that were diagnosed with breast cancer, just like me. Feeling the need for connection, I signed up, attended, and then kept attending. It literally changed my life. I gained strength, hope, and support from others that spoke my same language, that understood my timeline of Time before Cancer and Time after Cancer. I met with people that understood me and what I was going through better than anyone else. I sat in weekly, with skilled leadership and facilitators that directed and redirected topics of concern brought to our group. I shared my story: The diagnosis, treatment, my recovery, my fears, and my joys within that group. I learned in that group because we all built each other up. We all sharpened and embraced each other with our transparency while we participated, battled, and healed. I have new friendships that were fostered during that time, and we continue to support each other even now.

From the Lunch Bunch, I eventually promoted to the Wellness Group. The Wellness Group was great—it was weeks of sharing the aftermaths of our journeys. It was strengthening our bodies through Yoga. Special presentations by guests shared information about nutrition, intimacy with our partners, family dynamics, life after we return to work, and more. CSCP has left the light on for me! I now enjoy nutritional seminars, updates, and special events occasionally, even if I don't need the regular support to the extent that I got it before.

At one point, I could have chosen to take the elevator from my work office to the 2nd floor for in-house Yoga, but I chose instead to get in early and leave early to attend CSCP's Yoga offering that was sensitive and specific to my journey. My job has a club called LIFE: Women struggling with and beyond breast cancer. Once, when the ladies got caught up in the woes of treatment, recurrences, fear, darkness, loss of self-esteem; I modeled what I learned from CSCP's facilitators: "So...after you cursed God, your husband, your best friend, and your medical staff, what did you do? How did you pick yourself up and make it here today? What has anyone else done to get through those moments?" This is how I pay it forward! I needed those words of wisdom when I was still in the trenches, and now, I lock arms with other women as we continue to move forward and beyond cancer.

At the end of each Lunch Bunch session, we were given the opportunity to share a thought. My common share was just two simple words: Hope floats! Cancer Support Community continues to give hope, not just for breast cancer patients, but for all that fall under the cancer umbrella. It is there so that no one faces cancer alone.

I've taken my faith and CSCP and made them my tools. I've declared that cancer can't get rid of me! Fear is a huge factor that grips you when you hear those words for the first time, and many people wallow in a dark place after hearing them. But rest assured that you are not required to remain there. You have options! You are important. Your battle is important. Your story is important.

INTRODUCTION

"You have breast cancer."

The four words that can change the course of any person's life forever. Even after you recover, life is never quite the same. Something about cancer is vastly isolating—you feel like you are living on borrowed time, or like the life you once thought you had is one you no longer have.

This is true—once you hear those words, you know that life will no longer be the same. However, life does not have to be miserable. Life does not need to feel hopeless or impossible. Life does not need to be so incredibly terrifying that you don't know how you will go on.

Remember this—you don't have to fight your cancer alone. Yes, you will have your team of people there to help you—your support built upon the community, the medical professionals, and everyone else. However, you also have access to endless resources. Lean on this resource in your time of need—let this book be a helpful guide to figuring out what it will take for you to get what you need the most. This book takes all of my own experiences, what I learned, how I learned to fight, and how I survived to ensure that I got through my own journey.

Now, every person out there will have a journey that looks a little bit different. Some people's cancers are treatable. Some are not. Some catch it early, and others catch it when it has spread too much to treat. No matter where you fall with your own experience, however, know this: You don't have to fight alone. You don't need to be without support.

Within this book, you can hopefully answer some of the biggest questions probably going through your mind. You will learn what to expect over time. You will learn more about cancer and what it is. You will learn about how you can keep your strength up as you cope with cancer and get treatment. After all, treatment can be brutal, but maintaining your body in some form or another can make a huge difference. We will look into healthy foods that can help to gently nourish your body—we will look at tried-and-true choices for many women suffering from breast cancer that claimed that the foods were more palatable, easier to stomach, or just easier to enjoy, even when chemotherapy or radiation leaves them nauseous.

We will also look at the emotional side of things, looking at how intimacy with your spouse can be greatly affected by this process and treatment, and yet, is something that is highly important for you and your relationship to continue to focus on. We will look at how you can work to maintain that spark and intimacy with each other, even when you don't feel like you want to be physically intimate. We will also consider the changes to the family dynamics during this time in your life. Things change when you are diagnosed, and understanding those changes is a great way for you to learn how to cope with them better. Finally, we will look at how life looks and what to expect when you return back to work. It can be a trying time; trying to learn how to exist in this new normal for you can be draining, but it has to happen—it must be done.

Think of this book as your own personal guide to everything that you will need to know about surviving through the unthinkable. It's difficult to let yourself feel like you can get better. It's difficult to cling to the idea that everything will be just fine at the end of the day. However, mindset is everything when facing down an enemy like breast cancer. Mindset drives you forward—it will help you remain firm, help you have that resolve to fight.

Remember, you do not have to give up. You are a survivor. You are a warrior. You have the power to fight within you if you are willing to take it. Take that moment to curse the world, and then get right back to doing what you are meant to do—survive and thrive.

CHAPTER 1:

What Is Breast Cancer?

When I was first diagnosed with breast cancer, I knew little about it. Prior to being told those words that changed my life, I didn't think it mattered much—it was an invisible enemy that would not impact my life, and as such, I never bothered to really learn much about it. I've learned over my years this is not abnormal—many people who have no reason to learn about the ins and outs of cancer are entirely clueless when it finally becomes relevant.

Against best practices, when I was first diagnosed, I immediately turned to Dr. Google for a second opinion. I wanted to know everything that I could about that cancer to be prepared—even if that meant that I had to navigate through the potential false information. Thankfully, I did receive the information and answers to every question I eventually had thanks to my medical team. In particular, I had the support of my physician's assistant, my surgeon, my plastic surgeon, and my social worker. They all educated me and worked with me, teaching me everything that I needed to know or wanted to hear about my diagnosis.

I learned while every diagnosis is unique—every diagnosis comes with its own symptoms, its own changes, and its own general treatment. In my case, my first noticeable symptoms were pain and blood spotting from the nipple. However, for some people, they may be entirely asymptomatic when it is first caught. Others may find they notice a change to the shape of their breasts or a lump they can feel underneath the skin that wasn't there before.

I was diagnosed and in treatment planning just prior to the beginning of Breast Cancer Awareness Month with both diagnoses. This meant that I had access to awareness from many different messaging venues, seminar offerings, blogs, and other sources, all readily available. I felt very fortunate to have these options for learning and awareness in my face.

That's where this chapter comes into play. This chapter is here to guide you through understanding what breast cancer is, where it begins, and how it will affect you. When it comes right down to it, knowledge is power. Knowledge will help you to ensure that you can get through this. Arm yourself. Become aware of what you can do and what you can control and accept what is outside of your control. The content of this chapter is information found on **breastcancer.org** as well as the American Cancer Society. Time to get your learn on!

Breast Cancer Defined

Breast cancer is just one of several kinds of cancer that people can suffer from and requires a medical diagnosis. It is cancer that begins in the breasts, as the name implies. As cancer grows in the breasts, it creates masses that can either be visual on imaging, or it can be felt as a lump. It is almost entirely specific to women, but cases are documented of men who have suffered from breast cancer as well.

Cancer itself is something that many people don't understand. It is caused by cells that grow out of control. They are cells that stop growing and dying normally, causing problems. It can often be treated for people, but it depends highly upon the type, the stage, and the location of the cancer among a myriad of other factors.

Cancers, no matter the kind of cancer it is, are all alike in the sense they are cells that are no longer dividing properly. The cells within our bodies all have very specific jobs, and usually, when they exist, they grow, work, divide, and die according to their blueprints. This allows your body to function over time. However, when cancer starts, the cells grow beyond that point of a loss in functionality; they continue to grow despite the programming telling them to stop, typically due to either damage to the cells or due to mutations in the cells that happened during division at another point in time. The problem that causes is that you now have cells dividing rapidly when they aren't supposed to, and very quickly because they are not programmed to kill themselves at the point of malfunction, they spread and divide more and more.

Over time, they crowd out the cells that are supposed to be there—they take over the area, causing problems and potentially even spreading. When cancers spread from one region of the body to another, infecting an unrelated body part, it is said to have metastasized—the resultant tumors are metastases. Cancer that spreads from your breasts to your brain or bones is still the same cancer from the breasts, hence it is still considered breast cancer. Cancer is named after where it has started, not where it ends up later on.

In terms of cancers, they all vary greatly. Some grow quickly or readily spread. Others grow slowly and are highly responsive to treatment. Some are treated well just with surgery, while others require the use of chemotherapy, or even several treatments.

Ultimately, depending upon the type of cancer that you have, it will have its own treatment method. Your doctor will help you to discover the right kind of treatment for your specific situation to ensure that you have the best chances of defeating the cancer.

Where Breast Cancer Begins

Breast cancers begin from different parts of the breasts. Where the breast cancer starts is typically referred to in the type of cancer that has been developed. Breasts are complicated body parts—they have the ducts that carry milk, and they have the glands that will make milk. There are also other tissues in the breast that can develop cancer as well. If you have cancer in the breast, it will typically be one of several types.

Beyond just identifying whether the cancer is in the breast, it also must be defined with whether it has started and remained localized in one area, or it has spread or invaded surrounding tissue. This is referred to as either in situ or invasive breast cancer. In situ cancer has not yet spread—it is, for example, cancer that has grown in one type of tissue, such as in the duct or in the gland. If it is only in the duct, it has not yet spread and, therefore, would be in situ. If it has infiltrated the surrounding tissues, it is referred to as invasive.

I was diagnosed with ductal carcinoma in situ—DCIS. This is cancer that has developed in the ducts without spreading outside of it. It was caught early, before it could invade the other parts of my breast or body. Ductal refers to the fact that my cancer formed in the milk ducts. Lobular cancers, on the other hand, start in the glands that create breast milk. There are other forms of cancers that are less common as well, but can be just as terrifying to cope with.

Remember that although breast cancer is normally noticed due to lumps in the breast, not all lumps are actually dangerous. Percentages suggest that, if you find a lump in the breast, it is more likely to be benign than not. Lumps can be caused by things other than underlying diseases. If you are reading this book because you are worried that you have cancer despite having not yet been checked, it is normal to be scared, but it is always best to schedule an appointment with your care provider. And, if the lump is cancerous, please remember that early detection can save your life.

Stages of Breast Cancer

Once breast cancer has been diagnosed, the next plan of attack is usually to figure out how to treat it, and that requires your medical team to understand what stage of cancer you are in. This refers to the characteristics of the cancer, how it is working within your body, and how it is likely to spread. Diagnosing the stage of cancer allows your medical team to understand how to approach the situation to be certain that you can get the best, most effective form of treatment possible.

Breast cancer is typically expressed on a scale from 0 to IV. Stage 0 is, as the name implies, not very advanced—it is usually relatively early into its development, and cancer usually isn't particularly aggressive at this stage. By stage IV, cancer has spread outside of the breast and has infiltrated other parts of the body.

To determine the stage of your cancer, your medical team will work to see if the cancer has spread. Usually, this is done during the surgery being done to remove the cancer, if that is the plan of attack for you. During surgery, your doctor will also look at the underarm lymph nodes, the point where the cancer is the most likely to spread, and will often order additional tests to visualize cancer if it is suspected elsewhere.

Stage zero

At stage zero, cancer is non-invasive. It is "in place". This is what I had—DCIS is cancer that has not spread to other parts of the tissue. This is the earliest stage of detection, and I was very fortunate to have identified it before it could spread.

Stage I

Stage I cancer is invasive—the cancer has begun to spread throughout the breast. It is invading normal breast tissue around the localized occurrence. Typically, you can expect this cancer to be broken down into stage IA and IB.

In IA, the cancer is noted to have a tumor measurement of up to 2 cm. And the cancer must be limited to just the breast at this stage—there should be no involvement with the lymph nodes at this point.

In IB, however, the cancer presents differently. It could either present as no tumor at all, with just small clusters of cancer cells at smaller than 2mm, but larger than 0.2mm within the lymph node, or it could be the case there is a tumor of less than 2cm while there are also small groups of cancer cells present in the lymph nodes as well.

If the cancer responds to estrogen or progesterone, it will almost always be defined as IA, regardless of the development. It is also possible for cancer at this stage to invade microscopically, but not more than 1mm in distance from the main tumor.

Stage II

In stage II, cancer is typically classified into categories known as IIA and IIB.

Stage IIA is typically used to describe invasive breast cancer that meets the following criteria:

- No tumor in the breast, but cancer of larger than 2mm is present in 1-3 lymph nodes in the arm or near the breast bone, OR

- Tumor is present, measuring 2cm or smaller and has spread to lymph nodes in the arm, OR

- Tumor is larger than 2cm but smaller than 5cm and has not yet spread to the lymph nodes at all.

However, sometimes, if the tumor is within the range of 2 to 5 cm and has not spread to the lymph nodes and is not responsive to hormones, it will still be classified as stage I.

In stage IIB, however, cancer is typically noted to have signs such as:

- The tumor is larger than 2cm, but smaller than5 cm and there are small groups of breast cancer of under 2mm found within the lymph nodes, OR

- The tumor is larger than 2cm, but smaller than 5cm and has spread to 1-3 lymph nodes in the arms or breastbones, OR

- The tumor is larger than 5cm but has not spread to the surrounding lymph nodes at all.

Stage III

Stage III is invasive breast cancer usually classified as IIIA, IIIB, or IIIC.

IIIA will show signs of:

- No tumor present in the breast, or tumor of any size, while also present between 4 and 9 lymph nodes in the arm, or near the breast bone, OR

- The tumor presents as larger than 5cm and groups of breast cancer cells are detectable in the lymph nodes, OR

- The tumor is larger than 5cm; cancer has spread to up to 3 lymph nodes in the arm or breastbone.

IIIB typically presents as:

- Tumor is of any size and has spread to the chest wall or skin, causing swelling or ulceration, AND

- It may have spread to up to 9 lymph nodes in the arms, OR

- It may have spread to lymph nodes around the breastbone.

IIIC usually is diagnosed based on these criteria:

- The breast may or may not have a tumor within itself of any size, and may have spread to the chest wall or skin, AND

- The cancer is in 10 or more lymph nodes, OR

- The cancer has spread to lymph nodes above or below the collarbone, OR

- The cancer has spread to lymph nodes in the arms or breastbone.

Stage IV

Stage IV cancer is any cancer that has spread outside of the breast and lymph nodes to infect other areas of the body. It may have infected the skin, the lungs, the bones, the liver, or the brain. These are some of the most commonly hit areas. Typically, at this stage, you hear that your cancer is advanced or problematic in other ways. It is important for you to understand that this cancer can still be treated.

How Breast Cancer Spreads

As the cells in your breast go haywire and create more cancer cells, it is possible for cancer cells to break off and infect the blood or lymph system, which then carries them away to infect other areas of the body. Typically, this works because the body is all so interconnected—those cells reproducing in your breasts can get dislodged and wind up planting themselves in a bone somewhere, and once there, they can then reproduce themselves.

If the cancer is going to spread, it will almost always go through the lymph system. This is the series of lymph vessels throughout the body that connect your lymph nodes—the little parts of your body designed to take care of your immune system. They work to filter out the byproducts and waste. When cells end up in your lymph nodes near the breasts, they are then usually carried away by the lymph fluid throughout the body.

Once the lymph nodes have been infected, there is a higher chance that those cells will then spread throughout the body, metastasizing and causing all sorts of other problems for you. Your doctor will be paying close attention to this to make sure that you get the treatment you need to give you the best fighting chance.

Treating Breast Cancer

For treating cancer, you primarily have three options that the doctor will talk about. All of these can seem intimidating at first, and for good reason—you can get surgery, chemotherapy, or radiation. None of those sound very appealing, do they? There is a reason that people fighting cancer are called warriors, and it is because the options available to you are so difficult to get through. Battling cancer—each option is difficult in its own way.

Surgery

Surgery is designed to take out the cancer that is present. Maybe the body part infected will be removed entirely; with breast cancer, this is typically in the form of a lumpectomy or a mastectomy. The cancer is removed, along with the body parts. This, of course, carries with it recovery time that can be difficult. It can also lead to other problems. An often-overlooked problem with getting surgery for breast cancer is that women feel like they are less of a woman when they no longer have their breasts in front of them. They feel like having their breasts removed is too drastic, and that can destroy their sense of self-esteem. Sure, it is possible that you can get plastic surgery to bring back a sense of normalcy, but those breasts you knew and loved, those parts of you that may even have nourished your children, are gone. An entire part of you has been removed, and because of that, you can struggle. This is understandable and to be expected. It is life changing. It is painful. It takes time to recover, and you may find you have huge emotions during this time.

Chemotherapy

Chemotherapy is the use of drugs to treat the body. It is typically given through an IV, straight into the vein through a needle to treat the cancer. The drugs will travel throughout the entire body through the veins, making it effective to treat cancer that is spreading. It works by effectively stopping or slowing the growth of cancer cells. However, it also harms other cells that are healthy and rapidly growing. It essentially works by killing off cells currently in the process of splitting in half. Because cancer cells rapidly reproduce, they are also rapidly dividing, meaning that chemotherapy can target it specifically.

It can also be given in pills taken, creating a very similar effect that can be used with no invasive IVs that require the use of medical professionals to manage.

Because of the treatment causing damage and killing cells in the process of dividing, it also causes effects on other parts of the body as well. In particular, you can expect to see side effects such as:

- Hair loss or lack of hair growth which is usually temporary and completely reversible when therapy ends. And while the case, please note that hair loss does not occur with all chemotherapy

- Lessened immune system due to bone marrow being damaged

- Problems with the skin and digestive system

Radiation

Though I was fortunate to not have to use radiation therapy, three of my sisters have used this treatment with high energy rays, that destroy cancer cells. Radiation therapy is used in many different situations.

- After breast-conserving surgery (BCS), to help lower the chance that the cancer will come back in the same breast or nearby lymph nodes.
- After a mastectomy, especially if the cancer was larger than 5 cm (about 2 inches), if cancer is found in many lymph nodes, or if certain surgical margins have cancer such as the skin or muscle.
- If cancer has spread to other parts of the body, such as the bones or brain.

The main types of radiation therapy that can be used to treat breast cancer are external beam radiation therapy (EBRT) and Brachytherapy, radiotherapy in which the source of radiation is placed (as by implantation) in or close to the area being treated. EBRT is the most common type of radiation therapy used for cancer treatment.

External Beam Radiation

Common among most women with breast cancer a machine is lined up outside the body focusing the radiation on the area affected by the cancer. Which areas need radiation depends on whether you had a mastectomy or breast-conserving surgery (BCS) and whether or not the cancer has reached nearby lymph nodes.

If you had no lymph nodes with cancer cells after the mastectomy then radiation is generally focused on the chest wall and places where any drains exited the body after surgery.

> **For more information about treatment options visit:** *https://www.cancer.org/cancer/breast-cancer/treatment.html*

No matter the kind of cancer you have, no matter the staging or the spread it has achieved, remember that you can fight. You can still work to keep it at bay. Remember that the best thing you can do when diagnosed is to be hopeful, make sure that you are following the recommendations of your doctors and the medical team that is there to support you. Talk it through!

It's tempting to go online and search for those fad diets and fad treatments that tout they are some sort of miracle cure—it can be so tempting to cling to literally anything to give you hope but remember—your medical team is there for you. A second opinion is an option for consideration and will often be a further stamp of approval and assurance of the treatment plan offered by your medical team.

CHAPTER 2:
WELLNESS EXERCISE AND ACTIVITIES

Regular exercise and wellness are important for all people, whether they have cancer or not. Our bodies are designed to move.

Some jobs can keep us inactive. We may sit at desks for long periods of time. When commuting, we drive long hours to get to and from work and other events. When we don't really get moving, unfortunately, that just adds to the overall lack of health we suffer from. Our bodies need to be used to keep them functioning, and when trying to fight breast cancer, it is even more important than ever to keep your body moving and as healthy as possible.

During cancer, you probably feel exhausted. You feel tired and worn down. The treatments, whether you receive surgery, medication, or radiation, are hard! Your body needs to heal, and naturally, you will want to settle down and rest. But, did you know that mild activity is actually *good* for the healing body? Your medical team after surgery will probably encourage you to move around as much as you can while you recover. Of course, you need to be mindful of your limitations, but the movement itself is healthy. It will help you to ensure that you are going to recover well. It keeps the blood pumping to heal the parts of you that need it the most.

When I was fighting cancer, I took classes offered at the CSCP—they offered all sorts of different classes tailored specifically to people suffering from cancer. The instructors were well aware of the challenges we faced as we fought a disease that, historically, has been a death sentence. It is no longer that—it is something that we can fight, and we can win against, and keeping our bodies active can help us with that.

My instructors were always incredibly sensitive to the fact that people with cancer typically are tired. We are in pain. We are often self-conscious, frustrated, or even feeling defeated. Cancer is draining for even the most confident of people to fight, and because of that, you need to find ways to help sustain yourself.

The great thing about exercise is that it helps in many different ways—it works with you to make sure that you are feeling your best physically and that you can treat yourself as much as possible. It works with you to keep your body functioning, even when you feel like other parts aren't. However, there is also a mental aspect to it. When you get out there and exercise, you are accomplishing something. You are doing something difficult, and those little wins can keep you moving forward. Those little wins will remind you that you can keep fighting—those little victories when you finally manage that new yoga pose you have been trying to accomplish or when you get a new best time on your exercise will help you to remain in the right mindset to defeat your cancer as well. The mind is just as important as treatment physically during this difficult time, and exercise can help you to maintain it.

Within this chapter, we will look at this more in-depth—we will be talking about how there are serious limitations in your movement at first when it comes to getting treated for breast cancer. We will look at the importance of getting up and moving, as well as how to keep yourself motivated. Remember, even a few steps a day is better than nothing. If you can't run a marathon, try walking a block. Anything is a victory, no matter how small.

The Importance of Movement and Recovery

As previously stated, regular exercise during treatment for cancer is incredibly important. Not only will it help your body to keep its strength up as much as possible during your treatment, but modern research is also actually showing that with exercise and maintaining health, you can lower the risk of a recurrence. While this doesn't mean you have a clear pass to avoid cancer in the future just because you have started exercising, you will probably want to do everything that you can to lessen your risk.

Beyond just helping lower risks, recognize the fact that exercise will also work to boost your energy levels, and there is a good chance that through this entire process, your energy levels will be low. This isn't something that you can help—the treatments and recovery are brutal. But, with exercise, you can keep your body accustomed to some degree of movement. You can help yourself to feel healthier and keep your body in the best shape it can be in, given the circumstances, through movement.

You need to be mindful of your own limitations. There are plenty of limitations during this time, especially because the cancer you are trying to fight against is located right in your chest—right around those muscles you use for functionality.

Exercising Safely

For being able to exercise safely, you will first want to get approval from your doctor. They will know where you are in your treatment better than anyone and can help to provide you with the best possible advice, considering the situation. Through using their judgment and remembering to exercise safely when recovering, you can help yourself greatly.

It is incredibly important that you are careful with yourself during this time. You may be at risk for swelling in the soft tissues in your arms, hands, or torso due to surgery or other treatments, and sometimes, that can come with numbness, which can pose a bit of a challenge if you are trying to exercise. You want to feel what you are doing to make sure that you are being safe.

Some exercises considered risky during your recovery and treatment include:

- Swimming laps that require arm movements—you could swim with a kickboard instead

- Resistance bands—these can stress out the arms and put too much strain on those muscles

- Inverted yoga poses—if you have to put weight on the arms, you should probably avoid it

- Elliptical—while these seem like an easy cardio source, they also will be too straining on the arms.

Before you start exercising, there are a few points to remember to make sure that you can keep yourself safe. Remember, you want to take all of the precautions necessary so you don't actually hold back your treatment instead of making it better. Follow these steps to keep yourself as safe as possible during this time without overdoing things.

1. **Have a conversation with your doctor:** Your doctor will always know best. Stop and ask him or her what the opinion is. Are you healed enough to begin exercising? Are there any movements, in particular, he or she wants you to avoid? Make sure that you understand all of the limitations before you begin.

2. **Take necessary precautions:** When you know what your precautions are, you will then need to follow them as much as possible. If you need to, consider making use of compression garments or gloves, especially if you have been diagnosed with lymphedema.

3. **Warm up first:** You want to make sure that, before you begin anything, your muscles are ready. Start by walking for a few minutes before exercise and then work on stretching out all of your muscles, with regard to any limitations set by your doctors.

4. **Slow and steady wins the race:** While exercising and getting fit can be a slow improvement when recovering from cancer you can expect the process to be even slower. Remember, your body is training. It is recovering. It is fighting. You can't expect it to snap back as quickly as it used to just because you want it to. Give yourself time and recognize that even a little bit of progress is still progress.

5. **Be mindful of form:** Remember that when it comes to doing more or keeping the form right, you want to practice that form. This means that, if you are doing yoga, you want to hold your pose perfectly instead of holding it for longer. This will help to make sure that your body is moving as intended instead of being forced to do something incorrectly.

6. **Pay attention to pain:** If it hurts, there is probably a reason for it. Exercise is not supposed to be painful, and if you notice it is, you should probably stop and ask your doctor.

7. **Rest often as needed:** If you find you are feeling particularly run down one day, give yourself the rest you need. Focus on getting healthy first —this means making sure that you are providing yourself with rest if your body needs it.

8. **Cool down:** Finally, make sure that after exercising, you always cool down and stretch. Walk another 5 minutes to let your body slow down to help it adjust. Stretch out all of those muscles again. Your body will thank you for it in the long run.

How to Motivate Yourself When You Really Don't Want to Move

Exercise can be difficult, even for healthy people. Not everyone is cut out for constantly wanting to exercise, even if it is good for them. However, you can work to motivate yourself! It can be tough, but it is *so* worth it. I joined groups to do yoga and that constant presence of other people also trying to recover and get treated really helped me to manage the situation and to keep myself motivated.

If you want to stay motivated, you can start by trying to set up a partner. Find someone you can join during exercise. While it's supportive to have your partner or spouse there, it can also be kind of frustrating sometimes to feel like you are constantly slowing down a healthy person. Your spouse may insist that it's fine and that they want to support you—but remember, this is about you and what you need, not what they need. To help yourself stay motivated, consider taking someone who is already surviving cancer with you on your exercises. Work out with someone who's already getting treated. You will feel a bit less self-conscious when you realize that the person you are with is also suffering similarly. It is easier to be open about limitations when you both know where the other is at.

You can also work toward goals you set as well. If you set goals for yourself, you can usually help yourself to achieve whatever it is that you want to do. If you want to work out four times a week, for instance, set a goal and help yourself to make sure that it happens. When you can keep up with the work and ensure that you are following the steps to achieve your goal, it's easier to stay on track. This is because if you have the plan out there and you know what you are doing, you already know what you need to do to continue. Imagine this—you have that goal of working out four days per week if possible, and you dedicate Monday, Tuesday, Thursday, and Saturday to the cause. Each day, you know that you will exercise. This now helps you to keep track. There is no mystery behind when you will exercise if you have told yourself that you will do so on those days every week. Now, you can't push off exercise because you know when to expect it, and that can help to keep that motivation flowing.

Of course, with a goal like that, you also need to be mindful of what you are doing and whether your body is currently in a position in which it can handle that kind of exercise. You will need to follow your body's lead, and even if it is your workout day, pay attention to the cues you are getting from how you feel.

Easy Exercises With Support

For setting up your exercise routine, you want to make sure that it is well-rounded. You want to make sure that you are getting your cardiovascular exercise while also keeping up with strength and flexibility. These are crucial for you to complete, and the sooner you do so, the sooner you can maintain that health you want to keep up with.

The American Cancer Society recommends 150 minutes per week of cardiovascular exercise with an additional 2-3 days of strength training every week. That can seem like a lot, especially at first, but remember that you don't have to be there immediately. Especially if you are still in treatment, be mindful of your limitations and work to those goals over time, little by little.

Let's go over some of the easiest forms of exercise you can do while recovering that will help you to stay strong and keep your body well, no matter what you are going through. Remember that you should always ask your doctor before starting any of these!

Walking

This is honestly one of the easiest ways to get your cardio in. Walk up and down the stairs if you have the strength to do so. Walk around the block. Even just walk across your living room if that is all that you can manage. As you exercise, your heart rate increases, and you can use that to help yourself stay healthy and strong. Walk whenever you can while also being mindful of your own limitations. Don't feel the need to push yourself just because you think that you can do more when your body is limiting you.

Yoga

This is one of the greatest, gentlest movements you can do that will keep your body healthy, and it is absolutely recommended as much as you can tolerate. Make sure that the yoga you are completing is gentle and it may be advantageous to find classes geared toward people recovering from various forms of treatment—they are there to help you heal little by little as much as you can, and they will be more mindful of your limitations.

Stationary bikes

Like walking, these are great ways for you to work to get some extra cardio activity without hurting yourself. You will primarily work your legs, meaning you are at less risk of damaging the areas in your body still healing. However, that's not a carte blanche to just continue to exercise even if you feel like you have hit your limit.

Exercise, but don't push yourself and don't punish yourself. Your body needs to treat itself.

Swimming

So long as you have no open wounds and your doctor has no objections, this is a great low-impact form of exercise. You will want to avoid using any arm strokes—but you can avoid those by simply using a paddleboard for that additional support, using only your legs to push yourself around. This is a great option for you to keep on moving without feeling the impact from other forms of cardio. If you want to treat yourself well and make sure that you are not wearing out your muscles or hurting joints that may be struggling under the pressure of treatment, this is a great option for you.

CHAPTER 3:

THE PROPER NUTRITION

All too often, well-meaning people would offer me advice about what I should eat to fight off my cancer. Didn't I know that I could use the Keto diet to cure my cancer? Why didn't I eat enough fruits and veggies? What about kale? Did I eat too many fast foods in my diet? The cancer must have been caused by GMOs! Many people had an opinion of what I was eating and how it influenced whether or not I had cancer.

The thing about opinions is, everyone has one, including me! But not everyone has a degree in nutrition, and all too often, those opinionated, well-meaning people think that they are offering you some miracle cure to your suffering—as if just changing the foods that you eat could actually fight off the cancer. The reality is, science doesn't support any diet as a cure for cancer. If it were as simple as eating certain foods, we would not have the cancer endemic that we do! Cancer is caused by genetic damage to cells that occur over time, and while some diets, especially those rich in antioxidants, can aid in alleviating some of that damage, they do not entirely prevent the occurrence of cancer. It is not a guarantee that if you eat a handful of blueberries and kale every day you won't get cancer, and in fact, so many people I know that have had cancer had it despite their own healthy diets.

Nutrition matters and your diet matters—but you also must be mindful of falling for those so-called miracle diets that claim to be the answer to all of your problems. You must make sure that you are eating foods that will actually help your body, but you can't let your diet be the only thing you do to keep your body healthy. A healthy lifestyle, in general, is imperative if you want to feel your best, and you can do that in all sorts of different ways.

This chapter will focus on the importance of nutrition during your journey. While it is not the only factor, it is certainly an important one. You need to ensure that you are doing everything that you can to keep your body well. Now, let's consider several points. It is necessary for you to understand how cancer and food are related, as well as the importance of a good diet during your recovery period in the first place.

We will also look at foods that are good to eat while fighting cancer—and if you look over the different foods provided to you in this book, you will see they are highly nutritious. They are filled up with all sorts of great vitamins and minerals that will help you to provide yourself with everything that you will need to keep yourself thriving. The food you consume sets the stage for your body; it determines how your body can respond. While they may not be the miracle cures, they still are a factor for keeping your body ready and armed with the strength to fight!

The Relationship Between Cancer and Foods

We can't quite point at foods and say they definitively cause cancer. However, through using observational studies, we can see there are definitely patterns between the consumption of certain foods and potentially getting cancer in the first place. There are foods that doctors know will put you at more of a risk of developing cancer later on, but that doesn't mean that diet is the determining factor.

The foods you eat are broken down by your body over time. Your body, in digesting them, releases free radicals—unpaired electrons able to damage the cells. They can damage the proteins and DNA in cells. Cancer, then, is caused in part by damage to cells over time. The more damage that your cells are exposed to, the more likely that you are to develop cancer in the first place.

Certain foods are known to be higher in free radicals—the more you eat of them, the more likely it is that you will develop cancer yourself. However, they are not definitive—you can't say that just because you ate a few cheeseburgers you got cancer. We all want to indulge sometimes, and that indulgence isn't responsible for your diagnosis.

Let's look at the foods high in free radicals likely to give you problems. These are foods you should mostly avoid in your battle against cancer and after. By avoiding these foods, you will find you lower (but do not eradicate) your chances of a cancer relapse.

Foods to avoid that are high in free radicals

- **Sugars and refined carbs:** These processed carbs are low in fiber and nutrition in general while being high in sugar. This causes a spike in blood sugar when you eat it, and that spike in blood sugar has been associated with breast cancer, among other diseases. Per the American Cancer Society, a diet high in sugar can lead to weight gain, which may increase the risk of breast cancer.

- **Processed meat:** Processed meats, such as deli meats, bacon, ham, and hot dogs can potentially increase the risk of cancer as well. According to the International Agency for Research on Cancer (IARC) it refers to meat treated in some way to preserve or flavor it. Processed includes salting, curing, fermenting and smoking. IARC is the cancer agency of the World Health Organization.
- **Overcooked foods:** When you overcook food, or even when you cook foods at high temperatures, you can end up with harmful compounds in the foods potentially linked to inflammation and cancer. In particular, processed foods and those that are high in animal fats and proteins seem to be the most harmful when cooked at high temperatures.

Now, remember—you could have a diet heavy in all of the above and never develop cancer. You could have a diet where you never set foot in a fast-food restaurant, and you eat nothing in the above lists and end up ill several times. The importance here is that you can increase or reduce the chances of getting sick in the first place. Think of avoiding these foods as allowing you to minimize your risk, a lot like how you would wear a seatbelt and have a car with safety features designed to prevent death in a car accident. You could have all the safety features in the world and still die in a car accident. There is no way to completely prevent that from happening, and likewise, we do not currently have a way to prevent cancer either. Consider eating healthy food during and after recovery, like taking the time to put on a seatbelt when you get in the car—you are giving yourself the best possible chances to survive and thrive.

The Importance of a Good Diet During Recovery

Treatment is difficult. It is uncomfortable, and your body needs the best fighting chance to make sure that it can endure everything that you are putting it through. No matter whether you went through chemo, surgery, or radiation, your body needs to recover, and you owe it to yourself to make sure that your body is as healthy as possible. The best diets you can eat are those that will provide you with all of the nutrients that your body needs. They are the diets loaded with everything that goes into them, from making sure that you are eating foods loaded with antioxidants, which aid in the removal of free radicals that will damage your body, to providing yourself with plenty of nutrients to keep your body able to repair itself, the food you eat matters—especially when you find you don't actually want to eat anything at all. Chemo, for example, makes people nauseous and that lack of appetite can make it difficult to eat what you need.

For making sure that your diet is wholesome, every bite you take counts. You must be able to eat the foods that will give your body enough energy to fight off the cancer. In particular, a good diet will have many great effects to help you not just heal, but also feel better in general. The right diet for your own cancer journey will have effects such as the following.

You will feel better

When eating the right foods to keep your body nourished, you may feel better overall. Your digestive system is loaded with probiotics—bacteria actually able to have a massive effect on your brain chemistry thanks to their ability to create neurotransmitters such as serotonin, a vital compound or element that helps fight off depression and anxiety among other conditions. Eating the right diet will help regulate that production to keep your mind balanced as well.

You keep your strength and energy levels up

When nourishing your body with all of the foods you need to eat, you will also find you can keep your strength levels up as well. You can make sure that your body has the nutrients it will need to build stamina and keep energy high.

You maintain your weight

Cancer causes weight loss in many cases. According to the American Society of Clinical Oncology, roughly 40% of newly diagnosed people report they had recently lost weight without an explanation. In addition, it has been found that up to 80% of people with advanced cancer lose weight. When you are ill, your body cannot work as effectively as it normally would, and as a result, you may discover that your body can start to weaken. You are not just losing fat when you lose weight—you lose muscle, too.

When you can keep your diet on track, however, you can sort of mitigate any weight loss associated with breast cancer. You can keep your body filled up with good proteins and healthy fats that will keep your energy levels up while building and maintaining your body.

You lower your risk of infections, and your body heals quicker

With your body running as optimally as it can, meaning it does not lack nutrients or calories, it can more effectively fend off infections. This is because when your body is nourished, you can heal quicker. Your body has everything that it needs to build up those new, healthy cells to heal your wounds and to fight off infection. This means you can recover from your treatments sooner with wounds closing and infections being warded off. While this won't always prevent infection, it lowers your risk. Nutrition experts have suggested Vitamin C, often found in citrus fruits also aid and contributes to prevention.

Foods to Eat to Nourish Your Body While Fighting Cancer and Beyond

Let me reiterate one last time—these foods will NOT cure your cancer! These foods will not be a guarantee you will not get cancer in the future. I wish I had a miracle food to offer you that would give you that benefit—However, we can discuss the food you should put an emphasis on during your treatment and after to help your body stay healthy. We have only one body—and those of us who have gone through cancer know that better than anyone else. We have one body we can nourish for ourselves. We have one body we can nurture to recovery, and that means we need to give it the best fighting chance to ensure that it is as healthy as possible. Let's look at the foods that will help you to remain healthy and strong now.

Proteins

Protein is essential for our bodies to function. It goes into our DNA in the form of amino acids. It repairs body tissues to help us create muscle and organs. It helps our bodies to keep our immune systems active as well. Protein deficiency leads our bodies to break down muscle instead—this is why when you don't eat enough, you lose weight in muscles. Because of how your body builds up muscle and can recover from illness or injury, you must provide it plenty of protein, and after chemotherapy, surgery, or radiation therapy, it is usually recommended that you up your protein content to help your body rebuild itself.

Here is a list of some of the best sources of protein you can use during your recovery.

- Poultry

- Fatty fish (salmon, tuna, etc.)
- Lean red meats (in moderation)
- Eggs
- Nuts and nut butters
- Beans and lentils

Fats

Fat gets a sort of bad rap most of the time. The thing about fat is that it is actually a very important part of a balanced diet. It serves as a highly potent form of energy that your body can use. Through breaking down fats and using them as a source of energy, your body basically has a backup source for all of its energy needs. However, not all fats are made equal. Choose in moderation.

These fats are quite beneficial—they can provide you with heart-healthy fats that your body will depend upon to heal effectively. These healthier oils include:

- Olive oil (extra virgin)
- Canola oil
- Peanut oil
- Sunflower oil
- Safflower oil
- Corn oil
- Flaxseed oil
- Many fatty seafood sources, such as salmon

Carbohydrates

Your body relies on carbs more than anything else as its primary source of energy. These carbs give your body the energy it needs to just exist. Carbs are also usually given a sort of bad reputation because people usually associate them with sugars. They *are* sugars, but there is a huge difference between eating a teaspoon of sugar, versus eating five strawberries, which bring to the table plenty of other nutrients as well. Carbohydrates themselves are not inherently unhealthy—and in fact, often, we eat all sorts of foods that are still high in carbs that are also nutritional powerhouses.

When feeding yourself, then it is important that you give yourself quality sources of carbs—you should be able to provide yourself with all sorts of sources of carbohydrates also loaded up with fiber and nutrients. The best sources of that come from fruits, vegetables, and whole grains. When you eat these, you are getting pure forms of nutrition, loaded up with everything that you need to stay healthy long-term.

These other sources of carbs bring with them fiber, which is good for your body. They are loaded up with insoluble fiber, which allows your body to push along waste without much of a problem. When you can push along that waste, you can then eliminate it. The soluble fiber binds with water, allowing that stool created to remain soft enough to make its way through the digestive system. If you need some ideas on carbs to enjoy during your treatment, consider:

- Whole wheat breads and pastas
- Sweet potatoes
- Whole grain rice (brown rice)
- Enriched cereals
- Peas
- Beans
- Fruits
- Vegetables

Water and liquids

Your body needs water to function— up to 60% of the human adult body on average is water, after all, and you need that to maintain your body's health and wellbeing. Blood is 50% water. Your brain, 80-85% and heart 75-80% water. Your lungs are 75-80% water content. Your skin comprises 70-75% water. Your kidneys, 80-85%

and muscles comprise 70-75% water, and even your bones, the hardest part of you, comprises 20-25% water. (Medical News Today) Your body needs water to work properly, and when you don't get enough, things start to go wrong.

When your body loses water, due to vomiting or diarrhea, or if you just can't bring yourself to bring in enough water, you can suffer from dehydration. When this happens, your entire body ends up all out of whack. Your body won't be able to function properly, and you will feel worse than before. Water is essential for you. Any liquids you consume can count and help to keep you hydrated, and health authorities commonly recommend eight glasses of 8 ounces of water every day, more if you are suffering from vomiting or dehydration. This could vary depending on your personal situation.

Vitamins and minerals

As you go through treatment, you also need to get plenty of vitamins and minerals to maintain functioning as well. This is in all sorts of forms but is most often found naturally through the foods you eat. You can buy them as supplements, but ideally, you would make sure that you are carefully adding in all of the vitamins naturally through eating food. You would make sure that you are eating a balanced diet, even if just doing so is something that is difficult for you.

Vitamins and minerals are most highly present in fruits and veggies in their densest forms, and you will want to make sure that you are eating these regularly. Generally, you want to make sure that you eat foods of all different colors every day as they typically have very different nutritional contents to them in the first place. This means you need to provide yourself with plenty of options you can eat.

If you find you are remaining nutritionally deficient even trying to be mindful of what you must eat, it may be worth it to speak to your doctor and ask them for recommendations on how to keep yourself healthy and which vitamin and mineral supplements may be right for you.

Antioxidants

Now, let's talk about antioxidants. We have mentioned these several times now. These are enzymes or types of proteins that act as catalysts for reactions that are able to absorb and attach to the destructive free radicals that may be present in your body. They are usually used to allow for the body to prevent the free radicals present to be removed. This gives them the benefit of protecting the cells in your body and, therefore, reducing the risk of cancer and cancer spread.

- When you want to consume antioxidants, the best sources are in all sorts of fruits and veggies, though it is also present in other forms. Remember that antioxidants are not always recommended in dietary supplement form, and you will want to talk to your doctor to figure out if this is right for you. However, eating healthy fruits and veggies can be great natural sources. Foods full of antioxidants include:
- Blueberries
- Strawberries
- Kale
- Beans
- Dark chocolate
- Dark Leafy greens
- Carrots
- Dark green veggies
- Sweet potatoes
- Potatoes
- Nuts
- Green tea
- Whole grains

- Extra virgin olive oil
- Fish

How to Eat Well When You Don't Really Want to Eat

For keeping yourself eating well, then you have a few options for yourself! You can make sure that you are choosing foods that will give you the best boost toward making sure that you are healthy. If you are mindful of your food choices, even when you feel nauseous and uninterested in eating, you can help give your body the best start it will need to stay healthy and keep yourself feeling great. Let's go over some recommendations now.

Make healthy choices

Your cancer treatment is not the time to go on a binge diet where you suddenly eat only cabbage soup or restrict calories. You should not be intentionally depriving yourself of healthy foods during this time. Instead, you should be making it a point to make good, healthy choices. Focus on keeping your diet balanced. If you need to, keep a list of the foods you are consuming regularly. This sort of diary for your foods will help you to see if you are falling short anywhere with your diet so you can make the necessary changes to keep yourself healthy. Some of the best healthy choices you can make include:

- **Favor whole grain over processed versions:** If you are reaching for the pastas, consider giving yourself the whole wheat versions instead of the plain white ones. The change from using enriched bleached flour to using flours that are whole wheat gives you more fiber and nutritional value.
- **If you're not hungry, try using juices:** Sometimes, it's easier to sip at juices all day instead of actually eating food. While you need to get your fiber in somewhere, this is a good way

for you to at least get those vitamins and minerals into your diet.

- **Make your plate half fruits and veggies:** When eating, half of your plate should be dedicated to fruits and veggies, with the remaining half being split between selected whole grains and protein.

- **Go meatless:** A few times a week, try to skip the meat altogether. While meat can be good for you, it is also good to give your body a bit of a break as well.

- **Eat salads:** Unless expressly told to avoid raw foods, try to include salads with your dinner to get in those rich greens with all of the vitamins and minerals they provide.

- **Limit sugary foods:** You can have fruits and veggies, but added sugars should be limited. Now, if all you can stomach is ice cream after chemo, there is no harm in that—getting something into your body is better than not eating anything, but if possible, try to cut back on the foods that are calorie-dense without providing much in the way of nutrition.

- **Choose lean meats:** Make sure that you prefer lean meats and fish whenever possible over fatty meats and try to keep processed meats to a minimum.

Eat even when you're not hungry

One of the more common side effects of cancer treatment is a lack of appetite. Some of the treatments can interfere with how food tastes. Some can lead to problems with just feeling hungry, or even being too nauseous to keep food down. If you find you are often not hungry, there are still ways you can keep your body nourished without having to worry so much about eating more food.

- **Reach for the high-calorie foods:** Depending on your tolerance for food during treatment, you may not want to eat much. You have to make those calories count. You will want foods not only nutrient-rich but also highly dense in calories as well to make sure that you give your body what it needs. Foods like avocados, beans, and nuts, are all very nutrient-dense and high calorie, meaning you won't need to eat as much of them at any point in time.

- **Eat a little bit throughout the day:** Spread out your consumption, so you never feel uncomfortably full. It is usually easier to tell yourself that you will eat a small snack when you aren't hungry than it is to convince yourself to eat an entire meal. Smaller meals that are nutrient dense can help with tolerance of food and get the nutrients needed.
- **Don't wait for hunger:** Similarly, eat at specific points, scheduling it in rather than waiting for hunger to strike.
- **Tempt yourself:** If you must bribe yourself with your favorite junk food, then do it! You should be eating healthily primarily, but no one will fault you if you go for that smoothie or pasta plate after treatment.

Use healthy foods to ease side effects

Finally, if you are suffering from side effects making it difficult for you to want to eat, there are ways you can ease that as well. Cancer treatment is uncomfortable, but with skill, you can bring it back to some sort of comfort level with the foods you are eating, so long as you are mindful of what the problem is and how you can treat it.

- **Constipation:** This is a really common side effect that no one likes to talk about, but you can treat it with foods relatively easily most of the time. Make sure that your diet is high in fiber, such as beans, veggies, and fruit. Also, keep water in your diet heavily.
- **Diarrhea:** Another common side effect on the other side of the spectrum is diarrhea. When you suffer from diarrhea,

you can bring relief by sticking to foods that are bland and keeping water handy. You will want to use foods such as bananas, rice, apples, and toast (BRAT foods) to keep your stomach full without upsetting it. BRAT foods aid with stool formation, reducing the loose watery stools from diarrhea.

- **Dry mouth:** Dry mouth is incredibly unpleasant, and if you aren't careful, it can lead to damage to the mouth as well. You can treat this, however, with pureeing your foods so they are easily swallowed, or choose foods naturally softer and liquefied already. You can always moisten foods by adding water, milk, sauces or gravies.
- **Nausea:** If you are suffering from nausea, you can treat it similarly to how you would diarrhea. You can manage the nausea by avoiding foods that are greasy or strongly flavored, and you can keep your foods bland with mild smells, while still maintaining plenty of water in your diet.

CHAPTER 4:

INTIMACY WITH YOUR SPOUSE

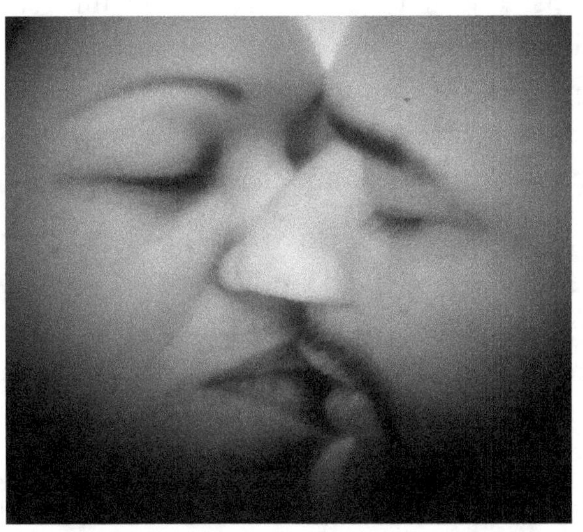

When cancer comes into your life, it impacts the life you knew before, and the life you knew before may cease to exist. So many things in your life are changed, affected on levels you never knew were possible. Perhaps the one tested the most is your marriage.

Cancer becomes the ultimate test of your marriage vows of "In sickness and in health." That diagnosis can change the one relationship you thought would never be changed.

When diagnosed, you suddenly have so much more going on. You have all sorts of doctor's appointments and treatments to go through. You may go from being a, presumably, able-bodied individual to suddenly needing help in even basic tasks you never thought that you'd be unable to do. You may be recovering from surgeries that will require you to go easy on your upper body for a while, meaning there are all sorts of movements off limits. You may be struggling to keep that sense of normalcy in other ways as well. Suddenly, foods you once loved become difficult to keep down, and your normal responsibilities now seem like insurmountable mountains in front of you that you can't handle. None of this is your fault, and it isn't your partner's either—but things may change, whether you want them to or not. Your partner will have to help more just by virtue of being your partner. Your own interactions with each other could change as you continue to rely on your partner more and more for support—and that's to be expected.

My husband and I settled down as I healed. We stopped being as active as we once were, and spent far more of our time together without physical intimacy. During this time, he was reassuring and kind. He was there to remind me I was still the woman he married and that I am beautiful just the way I am, no matter the cancer. Through his support, I realized that cancer didn't make me ugly—it didn't change who I am as a person. I am still me, and he still loves me.

We spent much of our time cuddled up together and we watched a lot of different movies. Our new norm during my recovery was movie night with popcorn, and he was always willing to remind me he was just fine with the way we were. He loves me for who I am, after all, and we can get through this. He was my rock, even when I was at my weakest.

When I told him my fears, he was a great listener. That wasn't always something he was known for during our marriage and yet, he was there with it right when I needed him the most. He allowed me to cry and vent uninterrupted when I needed to, becoming the shoulder I turned to the most. Then, he would offer encouragement and prayers and ultimately, he ushered me to where I needed to be emotionally, mentally, and spiritually. I recognized that his transformation in character was just for me. That in and of itself was a form of intimacy that helped me more than I ever thought it could have. His empathy and concern on my road to recovery helped to nurse me back to health. He guided me on the journey, and in doing so, he took care to protect and help to heal my heart as well.

Over time, I regained a newfound confidence in myself. His closeness, his ability to encourage me, and his ability to foster our intimacy in new ways was exciting and sowed into the power of our relationship. Soft kisses, compliments, romantic comedies, adjusting and readjusting my pillows were just a few elements in our newfound intimacy, and to me, they meant the world. I wasn't broken or damaged or ugly. Looks fade over time. They're not permanent, but what's inside of me—my heart and personality—that was what my husband saw when he looked at me. For a while, when I looked in the mirror, despite my newly reconstructed breasts, I saw a sickly woman, infected with a dark and toxic disease. He saw his loving wife he had promised to love and honor for better or for worse, and I felt blessed in that way. He didn't see me how I saw myself and that was for the best. That helped me. That emotional intimacy, that ability to engage, and that unconditional love were my everything. And, as an added bonus, he was there to remind me of something that I hope you will also take to heart. Scripture in Psalms 139:14 says, "I will praise You because I am fearfully and wonderfully made; Your works are wonderful, I know that full well." Pretty encouraging and powerful statement!

Intimacy doesn't disappear when you are diagnosed with cancer and can't do the things you did before. It doesn't disappear just because you no longer have the energy or appetite for physical intimacy. It transforms. It becomes something new. You find new ways to feel close to your partner, sometimes in ways you may never have considered in the past, and through that, you can maintain and foster your relationship or marriage, even in the face of something as destabilizing as cancer can be.

Intimacy and Relationships

Now, most people mistake intimacy for sex and let's get one thing straight right now: sex can be intimate, but it is not the end-all-be-all determiner of the intimacy you have with your spouse. It is important, and it definitely helps with fostering that bond with each other, but you can do so in other ways as well. Intimacy is more than sex. Sex is sex, but intimacy is love. You don't have to love someone to have sex with them, and likewise, sex is not always intimate, but love is. It is powerful. It can endure tests, such as what happens when you are diagnosed with cancer.

Intimacy still matters in your relationship, and you need it. However, you don't need to feel like you have to have sex you don't want. You won't always want it, and you may feel like you are no longer beautiful, especially if you have your cancer removed surgically or if you have endured mastectomies. However, you *are* still beautiful, and there are ways to help with emotional engagement to remind you of that.

You can show your partner you still love them through being intimate in other ways. You can be intimate emotionally. You can offer little physical reminders you are still right there, paying attention, and wanting to be close. You can cuddle. You can find time to watch movies together. You can talk. All of these are ways to become intimate without the need for sexual activity.

How Cancer Changes Intimacy

Cancer can be a huge strain on relationships in part because of the change to sexual intimacy. The treatments must be strong enough to take out your cancer, and in return, your body takes some of that damage as well. Sometimes, they can even change how your body responds and functions when facing a desire to be physically intimate in the first place. You may feel undesirable, or you may feel like you are too weak or ill to actually be physically intimate. If your appearance has changed, you might feel afraid to show yourself, embarrassed, or ashamed of the changes that have occurred. You might be all puffy from edema, or you may have lost a massive amount of weight. You might be scarred, bruised, or pale. You may have lost your hair. However, no matter how you have changed physically, you are still you.

Your partner may pull away sometimes. They may feel afraid of what will happen next or unsure of how they can help you. They may feel helpless as they watch their life partner suffer through cancer and the ongoing treatments. Intimacy can struggle on both ends—if you still want to and your partner is hesitant, you can run into other problems as well.

In terms of physical intimacy, cancer can disrupt in two distinct ways—it can cause problems physically with no longer feeling like you want to be sexual or intimate because of the discomforts you are suffering through. It can cause problems psychologically—your fear and insecurities may make it difficult to feel like your partner even wants you in the first place. Through my experiences of attending sessions with a diverse group of women that were diagnosed and battled breast cancer, it is so important that you are honest and transparent in expressing what you are feeling surrounding intimacy in your marriage. Remember, communication will help you to bridge that gap.

Depending upon the treatments you will endure, there are all sorts of side effects that can affect how you are feeling. You may suffer from side effects such as:

- Low or nonexistent libido
- Pain during intercourse
- Onset of menopause
- Body image issues
- Loss of sensation
- Fatigue
- Vaginal dryness

These are even more pronounced if you are in the group of women who have elected or been recommended to have their ovaries removed at the same time due to family history or BRCA gene prevalence. If you do have these symptoms, there are treatment options for you. Remember that you can always talk to your doctor if you have found you want to continue that physical relationship,

Fostering and Rebuilding Intimacy

As your relationship changes over time, the intimate connection with your partner may be one of the most important things that keep you feeling like you can get through the treatment in the first place. It will take communication, connection, and teamwork, but you can maintain that intimacy in a whole range of ways depending upon how you and your partner want to address it. Let's look at some of the best ways you can work to balance out your intimacy.

Be patient

There is no rush in cancer. You need to remember that you can take your time. Go at your own pace and listen to your body as you do so. Give yourself time to adjust to your reality when you are fighting or recovering from cancer—there are all sorts of different ways that your cancer will be affecting you, physically and emotionally, and you can't expect everything else in your life to stay the same. You need to be patient with yourself. If you can't be as intimate as you want, or if you don't want to be, you are not alone, and you are not broken. You are healing and recovering, and that takes time.

Communicate regularly

During this time, communication is key. Good communication is necessary for all relationships and is especially crucial during a trying time like this. You need to be able to communicate. Communicate your emotions. Let him know how you feel. Tell your partner what is going on in your mind and body. Let your partner know your fears or reservations you have about sex, or make sure that you are talking to him about what it will take for you to feel more comfortable. If you are not comfortable at all, let him know that, too, and talk openly about what you need and how you feel.

Work together

Remember, your partnership is a team effort. Especially when that team is knocked off-kilter, such as when you are suffering from cancer and need to be able to get that treatment in other ways, you will need to be able to find other ways to work together. You need to foster that closeness and companionship, and that will also help to connect and maintain intimacy as well. Let your partner know what you need and respond to his own needs as well. In doing so, you will find you can actually get so much further in your relationship than you probably realized was possible.

Make necessary accommodations

If you are interested in pursuing a physical relationship with your partner, you can do that too—you just have to make sure that you are taking the time to actually accommodate yourself. There are all sorts of adjustments you may need to make. For some women, they need to change the position. Others may need to involve lubrication to aid the dryness that can come with treatment. This doesn't make you broken, but it deserves to be accommodated as much as possible to ensure that you can do as much as possible with your physical relationship.

Validate each other

feelings. You both probably have many different emotions swirling around; you probably both feel frustrated or hurt. You are probably scared or angry or worried about the future. You can really help with emotional intimacy if you and your partner will take the time to validate each other. Take the time to talk to each other, to really make it clear to each other that you care. When you do this, you are able to better your relationship over time. Empathize. Remind your partner you are there for them, even if you can't fix the problem.

Get to know each other again

Life after breast cancer is different. Your whole world is rocked, and you can't do much to fix that. However, you can make sure that you start all over again. Even if you feel like you want nothing to do with any physical intimacy, and that is your right, you can still work through establishing your relationship in other ways. Get to know each other again. Date each other. Cuddle and hold hands. Remind each other of your love. Touch, touch, and touch some more.

Speak to your doctor

If you are unsatisfied with your sex life, tell your doctor. Your team is there to support you, and they have resources they can use to help you. Sex is rarely brought up by the doctor if you don't bring it up yourself first. It can be an awkward conversation to have, but if you are truly unhappy, bring it up. Your doctor can let you know how your treatment may affect your relationship and offer you any suggestions to work with the dysfunction you may experience.

CHAPTER 5:
FAMILY DYNAMICS

When everything changes, the lack of control you feel—that sensation of spiraling out of control—is real and horrific at the same time. You suddenly find yourself on a roller coaster ride that is now your life, and you want to get off! It is terrifying to receive such a devastating diagnosis, and as you press forward, you watch that life—your life—change. It is so incredibly crushing, and the threat those four words, "You have breast cancer," presents to the vision you have for the future can be overwhelming. It can shake up the very hope and faith you have!

Our youngest son was in high school when I was first diagnosed. He was a sophomore, excited to get on his way. He has always been a great achiever, dedicated and diligent, but after my diagnosis, things changed. He struggled more in school. He couldn't focus as much. His grades were affected to where when he was applying for college, he had to justify why his GPA had dropped so much during high school. Understandably, he was devastated at my diagnosis, and I was devastated that I couldn't shield my not-so-little-anymore boy from the impact of this disease.

Things changed at home, and instead of my son focusing on school, he became driven to research everything while trying to balance academics, athletics, and church involvement. He desperately wanted to be able to cure me—he thought that he might find something online that we hadn't tried, or that my doctor didn't believe in that could have been that magical cure. I couldn't blame him—he had hope he could fix things for me. He didn't want to lose his mother, and I didn't want to leave him with that hole in his heart.

My son came at one point, ecstatic with the research he had found. He insisted that if I drank alkaline water, I would be healed. Of course, there are no miracle cures for cancer, and while alkaline water may have specific health benefits, I had to share it wasn't a substitute for my treatment plan. The ongoing conversations after that point were difficult as well. I knew he was well-meaning, and I knew that it was his way of coping with the pain.

We lived in a constant state of unknowing. We were in the unknown, not knowing what tomorrow would bring. We didn't know what would happen the next time I went to the doctor. Every time I felt ill or had a new symptom, we were nervous. Was it the cancer? Was that headache just a headache, or was it the cancer spreading? It was incredibly difficult, and not knowing it took a toll on my whole family.

I was so thankful to have the great community I was blessed with. They were there for me as my family dynamics shifted. My son, that same one in high school at the time, was surrounded by church, family, and a close-knit basketball team able to support him. We needed the help. I, the mother of my family and the one supposed to be the nurturer for my children and a partner to my hubby, was now in the role of needing to be cared for. That upside-down role reversal was difficult, to say the least.

The second diagnosis was, in many ways, worse than the first. On one hand, my husband and I were alone—our children were all out of the house for the first time, but we also couldn't help but worry about our youngest son's performance in college. After all, my first diagnosis had been a huge hit to his ability to focus. He couldn't keep his mind on what mattered—his schooling. Would he do it again? Would he struggle to do well in class and this new college experience, wondering how I was doing when he was out of state? He expressed that he was worried about this, as well. He ultimately worked on himself and remained focused. He often says that in witnessing how strong that I was, in holding on to my hope and faith in God, I helped him. However, it was a definite struggle.

During that second diagnosis, our older daughter had been living in Texas. She had her own wonderful life, thriving as a high-profile nanny and was incredibly happy with where she was. She was concerned as well during that second diagnosis, so much so she decided to come home to California, uprooting everything out of her own concern for my health. While I appreciated having my daughter home with me, I also felt like it was sort of a slap in the face—they were supposed to be spreading their wings and flying, and yet here I was, sick again and bringing my children right back to the nest.

The family dynamic changes rapidly when you are diagnosed with cancer. Everything flips over, especially if you are a parent. If you are a parent with young children, I'd imagine that it is even more difficult when you have children that are too young to fully understand the true degree of seriousness that comes with such a heavy diagnosis. But remember, the family is strong. The family unit is resilient, and you will be glad you have their support. There is a great degree of adjusting that goes into being diagnosed and fighting this disease, but the good news is, you can endure. It is hard, but you can make it! Your spouse has promised to love you in sickness and in health; for better or for worse, and when cancer enters the picture, it is absolutely in sickness and for worse. It will be testing. It will be difficult. But remember this—you are a fighter, and no one should fight cancer alone.

Adjusting to the Diagnosis and Treatment

After a diagnosis, there is always an adjustment period for everyone in the family, whether they are in your house or not. Schedules may have to be turned around so you can be taken to your treatments, some of which may leave you unable to drive yourself around. You may need someone to help to take care of you or to meal plan or pay bills. You may need house cleaners or other supports, depending upon the role you played in your family before diagnosis. A stay at home mother diagnosed with cancer, for example, may need to be able to outsource a good deal of her chores, depending upon how she feels and what she is capable of. This is difficult and can leave you feeling like all is lost. Some of us love our autonomy. We love doing things on our own without relying on other people, but that becomes next to impossible during treatment for cancer. Here are just a few ways that life can change when facing cancer:

- **A change in roles:** When you have cancer, roles often change. Your primary job is to get better during this time. Many days, nothing else matters at all. Someone else may need to deal with the chores you used to take on. You may see older children needing to pitch in more with chores, or a shift to the bulk of household duties falling to the other spouse.

- **A change in money:** When you are sick, money is high on the list of concerns. Cancer can not only reduce money in causing you to lose a job or be unable to continue working, but it can also be incredibly costly. Checking all available resources is advised.

- **A change in living arrangements:** Depending upon your situation, such as if you live alone, you may need to move in with family or friends to get the extra care you need. You may need to move closer to your treatment location. You may simply not be able to afford your prior living situation when you have to also pay for the cancer treatments.
- **A change in daily activities:** You will probably find that many basic tasks you used to do regularly are now difficult for you after treatment. You might need someone to help you to take care of the pets, the dog for a walk or kids to the park. You may need help with all sorts of different activities, and you will need to acknowledge that.

Accepting Help

That brings us to the point of accepting help. You may be the most independent woman on the planet, a single CEO mom of three who runs a massive corporation who doesn't need to ask for help from anyone, but if you get cancer, that all changes. Cancer weakens your body. It makes you tired. Your treatments cause injuries that must heal. You are fighting off a dark and toxic disease. It's only natural you will need help.

And that's okay.

You should not only accept help when someone offers it to you, but you should also *ask* for it. Yes, it will change dynamics. Yes, it will put you in a position of vulnerability. However, you need to give yourself time to heal as well. It is not a sign of weakness to ask for help, and you will probably find that anyone that cares about you will be willing to give that help without much of a pushback. You just have to be willing to ask in the first place.

Remember that if you need it, you can also *outsource* activities. You can make sure that you are asking other people to take care of tasks you can't. Allow your family or circle of friends to set up a meal train to bring you food to alleviate that worry from you while you recover, especially after surgeries or other particularly difficult procedures. My co-workers planned a calendar and provided healthy home cooked meals while I recovered. Family, friends and my church community showed up! I am forever grateful.

Your Marriage or Partnership and Cancer

Your partner or spouse will be highly affected by cancer. No matter how solid your marriage is, this is perhaps, one of the most trying things you could go through—if an advanced stage of cancer you are facing what could well be a life-threatening disease. This can have a significant impact on your marriage in many ways. Stated previously, you and your partner may need to shift roles. If you have a husband who usually works while you stay at home with young children, there will be a massive shift in the dynamic between the two of you, and that can cause some serious adjustments. The most common changes in your relationship you are likely to face while fighting cancer include:

- **Changing roles:** When facing cancer, you will be put into a dependent role. You might not be able to drive or support or provide help with what is happening during the day. You may realize that you are not in a position of pushing the family further during this time—you are in a position of leaning on your family to treat and support you. You may notice that your partner tries to help by constantly researching the disease and trying to manage your treatment schedule. You might notice he errs on the side of being controlling in an effort to be helpful, and is well-intentioned.

- **Changing responsibilities:** Most relationships involve a divide in chores that is relatively unspoken—you may agree that you handle the dishes and the laundry while your partner cleans the floors, manages the lawn, and takes care of pets. It is pretty typical to have a divide like that, but if you find you are tired or too ill to move, your partner will naturally be the one that must pick up the slack somewhere along the way. You may notice that your partner is struggling to cope with that, but it is also not your fault either. Talk about this with your partner and figure out ways to fix those frustrations so they don't weigh so heavily on your partner that resentment breeds.

- **Physical needs change:** When you are sick, you can't help it—you must be able to meet your needs, but you might need help to do so. You might need help getting dressed or washing and brushing your hair and teeth after surgery, for example. It might be difficult to walk up the stairs. However, your partner is there as a support for you. Talk openly and express what you need.

- **Emotional needs change:** Your emotional needs will be incredibly important during life with cancer, as well as after. You will need to make sure that you and your partner both mutually check in with each other regularly to make sure that you are on the same page and that you are both taken care of as well.

Children and Cancer

Your children will notice that life has changed when you have cancer. There is no way around it—when you are diagnosed, everything will become different. You will need to be prepared for this and be ready to help with it as well. Your children will need you to be prepared to help them understand this tumultuous time in your family's life, whether they are adults already or still young and in your home. We are going to first look at the most common challenges you may face, the changes you will see in behaviors for your children before exploring how to balance those needs between yourself and your children.

- **Troubles with communication:** When it comes down to it, you need to be able to communicate with your children. You might want to protect them from being afraid of what is going on, but at the appropriate time, plan to explain what is going on and how things will change. Your child knowing the truth of your battle will be beneficial to all involved, and your children will appreciate feeling like you are trying to keep them informed and involved.
- **Changes to behaviors:** When your children learn about your diagnosis, they may show signs of their own behaviors changing. Some younger children will become clingy. Older children and teenagers may completely withdraw from the family. Both of these are normal ends of the spectrum, but remember that despite this, you should attempt to keep schedules and communication as consistent as possible.
- **Adult children and cancer:** If you have adult children, as I did, you may discover that, whether you intend to do so or not, you end up with a role reversal. When you have cancer, you need help. Your adult children, or even teenage children still at home, may become your caregiver. They may need to drive you places or pick up the groceries. They may need to make time to help you with extra chores around the house as well. This is difficult on both ends, but it may be necessary, depending upon your situation. That's okay. Be patient with the role reversals and the struggles that may come with it.

CHAPTER 6:

LIFE AFTER RETURNING TO WORK

Perhaps one of the biggest differences between work before and after cancer is the changes you encounter. It is difficult when every part of your life appears to differ from what it once was. When you are constantly struggling to cope with the changes to your life, you probably feel like you need some sort of stability somewhere. You want something to remain the same, and you assume that work will give you that sense of normalcy. However, when you get to work, you realize that it's not the same. Even work, something where your responsibilities probably have changed little, will be different.

The greatest battle of all, however, is that within your own mind. I was very fortunate to have a supportive work environment, but not everyone is. Not everyone can claim that, and I recognize exactly how blessed I was. However, I still found there were all sorts of changes to be made. I found that some of my colleagues treated me differently. They wanted to engage with me in different ways, and at times, I felt like I was handled with kid gloves. I didn't want to be treated as if I would break at a moment's notice. I didn't want to be treated like I needed to be babied. It bothered me a little and I couldn't quite explain it at the time, but I was growing in this new norm and I wasn't sure what to do about it in the moment.

I appreciated the help, and it certainly made the transition back to work easier to handle, but at the same time, it was also stressful. It was a constant reminder I was not back up to 100%. Over time, I realized that I had a kind of post-traumatic stress disorder of my own. I showed up to work and tried to work as much as I could, but I was also very jaded about it at the same time. Life was different and I was different and in constant self-assessment in a much-needed new season.

I needed to find my own balance. I needed to come to terms with my disease, my battle. I needed to find that place so I could do better and be better. Continuing wellness with mind, body, and spirit matters. I needed to nourish myself. My body was healing, but my mind and spirit were still down. I needed to come to terms with that so I could return strong.

When you return back to work after treatment, expect things to have changed—because they did. But the attitude that you go into the experience with will matter greatly. When you go back to work, you can realize that you can boost your self-esteem. You can get back to work and remind yourself that you are more than just your diagnosis. You can move on with life and remind yourself that you have a purpose—you are valued as an employee, coworker and to some, a friend. You will also get to go back to work and enjoy human contact again. Life with cancer can be lonely, especially if the bulk of your social circle before was work, and the experiences you had during the day and getting back to work can help you with that. You can foster those good relationships again. You can make sure that you feel like you are well connected to others. You can find some sort of purpose for yourself.

The transition isn't always easy, even with the doctor's newfound approval, or recommendation, that you return to work. Though the most crucial recovery time has passed, your body is still healing and regaining strength, little by little and day by day. However, you can make that transition easier for yourself by remembering three things. Take it easy, slow your pace, and give yourself grace.

If you are thinking about going back to work, listen to your body and talk to your doctor and medical team about it. If they express concern it is too soon, heed that warning. If they are agreeable with that request, then great! Learn what your doctor thinks are your limits and keep them in mind. It is imperative to your healing you listen to what your doctor wants for you. When you do this, you can usually work with your place of employment to accommodate those limitations so you can work so it is safe for you while still allowing you to do your job.

Know that you have rights. Even with cancer, you still have certain rights that should be given regardless of your diagnosis. Legally speaking, the cancer diagnosis should not be a problem for you, but sometimes, it can be if your employer pushes back at what you have been doing and the uncertain and unpredictable that goes with the journey. Talk to your employer to make sure that you are accommodated.

Planning Your Return

Again, if you're ready to go back to work, you must first talk to your doctor. Are you physically as ready as you are mentally? The familiarity can be something wonderful to look forward to because it is indicative of life before cancer. It is life before things changed.

You want to go back to normal, and one of the easiest ways to ensure that you can do so is to return to work and prior wellness.

To go back to work, however, make sure that your doctor agrees that it is right for you based on your treatment plan and on the cancer diagnosis. Your doctor will determine when you can go back to work based on three key criteria. First, your doctor will weigh the long-term effects of the treatment you have received, trying to figure out if you are actually prepared to go back to work. Your doctor will consider the physical demands of going back to work as well, looking at what it will take to determine if you are actually ready and physically capable of handling the workload you will have. Finally, your doctor will determine the level of care you will need to accommodate accordingly.

If your doctor approves your plan to go back to work, the next best thing you can do is make sure that you are planning with your workplace. You must contact the Human Resources department and arrange it with them. This means you will need to discuss your limitations, if any, the timing, and any expectations.

What Are Reasonable Accommodations?

Remember that your employer is under no legal obligation to lower their standards to accommodate your needs. However, your workplace has an obligation to accommodate an employee with a disability unless it would be an undue hardship to make them. This means that unless you have an accommodation that would be dangerous, difficult, or expensive to do so, your employer should be reasonable about it. This means there are certain accommodations you should be able to expect to use without much of a problem. These include accommodations such as:

- Offering devices or equipment that are modified
- Restructuring your job requirements without eliminating your position
- Offering a modified schedule to accommodate for any further medical treatments or granting permission to work at home
- Reassigning you to duty at a simpler job that is within your abilities to complete
- Adjusting their policies to ensure that you can work
- Assuring the workplace is ADA-friendly (Americans with Disabilities Act)

If they are not willing to work with you, you may find that talking to HR is in your best interest. You may also find that going to your union can help you as well. Make sure that you fight for your rights and reasonable accommodation. You want to make sure that you are getting everything that you need, and you have a right to your job, making an effort to reasonably accommodate.

Adjusting to Work

In the return to work and wellness are new challenges. You might find you repeatedly get too tired to continue working, or that you might forget things more often. You might also need to take more breaks sometimes to accommodate everything.

You can make some small changes that will help you to cope better. You can make it a point to make some simple changes that will help you. While work is meant to be a great source of pride and confidence in yourself, it can also be difficult to cope with everything surrounding your adjustment as well as your return to physical wellness. You might find you are stuck with trying to cope with the pain, the fatigue, or even confusion that may come with treatment. Chemotherapy and radiation are not easy on the body, and your body will need time to adjust accordingly. Try making these changes at work to help accommodate everything:

- **Take breaks regularly:** Even if you take them more often than is normal or expected, this would be considered a reasonable accommodation. If you need to sit down regularly, then do so. Don't make yourself feel like you need to push yourself further than you need to.
- **Make lists and alarms with tasks:** If your mind is still a bit foggy from all of the treatments or traumatic surgery, you are not alone. However, this is easily manageable just by setting some simple alarms and lists to keep yourself on track.
- **Discuss things of concern with your manager:** If any concerns come up, such as your own performance or how those around you are treating you, mention that to your manager. Don't be shy—they are there to help you
- **Take breaks for doctor appointments or as needed:** You should be able to take days off that may not normally be allowed based on your contract. Your employer needs to accommodate breaks that need to happen.
- **Ask for an easier role temporarily:** As you recover, you can ask to take on a new job at work to help yourself meet expectations and lower your own fatigue.

Now, socially, you will face some different challenges as well. Socially, you may feel isolated while battling cancer. Especially if you have no choice but to stop working, you might struggle socially. Returning back to work isn't the simple solution you would expect it to be, either. Sometimes, your coworkers may be confused about what you can do, how much work you can do, and how you will be able to get along. They may be worried that you will not be able to keep up with the work to be done, and they will have to take on extra responsibilities to accommodate you.

Returning to work can be complicated—it can be difficult for you to figure out how to navigate the process with your coworkers, but realize that they are human just like you. While they may not be struggling with your illness, they are still affected by it. If you will need help—that could translate to them needing to help you. You must take extra days off—and that could become more work for them to complete. They might treat you with those kid gloves I talked about earlier, too, and baby you. No matter their response, you must figure out how you will navigate the situation.

Communication matters here. You will need to communicate clearly and effectively to help them see what you need to do and how you need to do it. Communicating effectively is the best way you can make sure that your needs are met. If they don't know why you left abruptly in the first place, you can try explaining to them what you are going through. You can let them know as much or as little as you care to share, and this can actually help you to maintain that bond long-term. But it is something that you must consider. How much do you want to lean on them? How much do you want them to know about what you are doing? How much do you want to explain? You technically don't owe them anything at all—but it can help to reconnect and get back on that same page again, and that can be a plus.

Remember, you are an important part of your workplace. You play an important role. When you can remind yourself that you are valuable too, even when struggling with your own abilities, or inabilities sometimes, you can help yourself integrate more smoothly right back into life with your coworkers. Your mindset matters here. Remember this.

CONCLUSION

I wholeheartedly hope that through reading about my own experiences, my own recommendations, and my own opinions, you feel a bit more comfortable with the idea of facing breast cancer. While it is never an easy battle to take on, it is the one you have been dealt, and as unfair as that may feel, remember that you are not alone. You have joined this club that no one ever wants to face, but remember—none of us asked to be there. You are joining a community of women who can be amazing resources if you allow them to do so. You are joining a group of women that are willing and able to provide you with insight, with support, and with genuine friendship that can last a lifetime.

Cancer is not exciting for any of us, and no one wants to face the changes that go into life when it comes. It tries our faith, our relationships, our families, our jobs, and more. But, one thing is for sure. When you come out on the other side, you will be stronger. You will be a fierce survivor, capable of taking on the world, no matter what it throws at you. You can take on just about anything, all because you will have had to test your courage to carry on.

You are not alone. You don't have to fight alone. You don't have to put on a brave face and carry on as if nothing has happened. Be real here—something *did* happen. You got cancer. It happens. Be strong and fight! You have the power within you to survive.

Having a positive mindset is powerful when fighting cancer, and if you can keep a lifted spirit of encouragement, you may discover that you can do so much more than you thought was possible.

Thank you for being here to read my story. I hope that as you listened or read through it, some of the fear of the unknown has faded away and that you have begun to feel more confident in how you will approach your own battle. If you have that diagnosis, take some time to grieve. It is okay to feel devastated, scared, confused, and angry. It is okay to feel like the world is crashing down around you, and it is okay for you to feel the way you do. It is *not* fair you have to join this team. It is *not* fair you have to cope with the anguish, the pain, and the entirety of your world being flipped upside down by your diagnosis. But you can get through it. You can tackle that treatment and move on. Find your rock— your faith, your spouse, your best friend, your parents, or anyone else. Lean on them. Let them carry you when you get weak, just as you would carry them when they need your help as well.

If you are waiting to hear back about that diagnosis, don't let the fear consume you. Take a deep breath. Pick up your head. Wipe away the tears of anger, of anguish, and of fear. Hold your head up high and straighten out your back. Tell yourself that you are a warrior. Tell yourself that you can win. Tell yourself that you are a fighter and that you are a survivor.

Believe those words with all your heart. Let them guide you as you continue with your own story. Find support groups local to you and online. Make the effort to go out and do something for yourself.

I'd like to add a special thanks to Nutritionist and daughter-in-love, Victoria Smalley for her assistance and Lamag Entertainment Group for producing this audio book and publishing the Kindle and print versions as well. In addition, I'd like to thank the Life, Care and Prayer groups from Fellowship Monrovia and Bethlehem Church,

Pasadena for their support in so many ways. Please write a review on Amazon to let me know how you like the book and visit with me at natalieksmalley.com. God bless you!

Remember this:

Hope floats!

Cancer Support Community (cancersupportcommunity.org/about-us)

Cancer Support Helpline: (888)793-9355

As the largest professionally led non-profit network of cancer support worldwide, the Cancer Support Community is dedicated to ensuring that all people impacted by cancer are empowered by knowledge, strengthened by action and sustained by community. It is a global non-profit network of 175 locations, including CSC and Gilda's Club centers, hospital and clinic partnerships, and satellite locations that deliver more than $50 million in free support and navigation services to patients and families.

So that no one faces cancer alone.

Community is stronger than cancer.

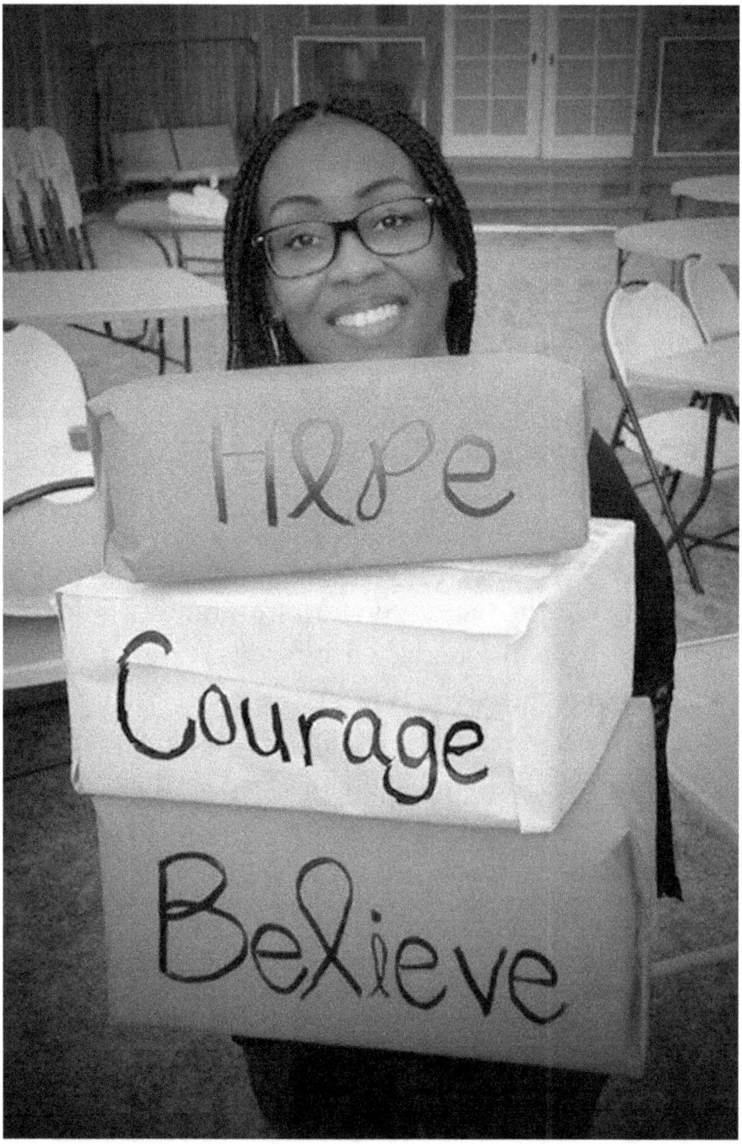

Natalie K. Smalley